Understanding Anal Fistula & Treatment

Treatment Odyssey and Exploring Options for Anal Fistula Management.

Title:
Understanding Anal Fistula & Treatment

Subtitle

Treatment Odyssey and Exploring Options for Anal Fistula Management.

Copyright © 2024 by (Dr. Joey Green)

Printed in the United States of America.

ISBN: 9798877159945

TABLE OF CONTENT

INTRODUCTION

Although many elements of our anatomy are well-known and understood, certain situations may be less recognizable to the general public. The human body is a wonder of intricacy, and while many aspects of our anatomy are well-known and understood. As an example of a condition that frequently falls into this category, an anal fistula is one example. In this detailed introduction, we will go into the deep specifics of what an anal fistula is, the numerous components of its genesis, and the fundamental necessity of knowing this ailment.

What is an Anal Fistula?

To begin our investigation, let's take a closer look at the word "anal fistula" to acquire a more profound comprehension of what it means. A tiny tunnel that arises between the surface of the skin around the anus and the inside of the anal canal or rectum is referred to as an anal fistula. The development of this aberrant connection often takes place as a consequence of an infection that occurs in an anal gland, which ultimately results in the production of a tract or tunnel. As a result of the fact that anal fistulas are frequently characterized by chronic pain, swelling, and discharge, individuals who are afflicted by them experience a source of discomfort and anxiety.

When attempting to explain the formation of fistulas, it is essential to have a proper understanding of the anatomy of the anal area. Several structures surround the anal canal, which is an essential part of the digestive system. These structures include the sphincters and the anal glands. An infection of an anal gland can result in the collection of pus, which can then lead to the creation of an abscess once it has been allowed to continue to grow. This abscess may produce a route or tunnel, which will result in the development of what is often referred to as an anal fistula if it does not drain correctly.

Importance of Understanding Anal Fistula

Although anal fistulas may not receive as much attention as many other medical disorders, they can still have a significant negative effect on a person's quality of life. The physical, psychological, and social components of managing anal fistulas must be acknowledged to fully appreciate their significance.

- **Physical Impact:**

Recurrent infections, as well as chronic pain and discomfort, can result from anal fistulas. For both patients and medical professionals, it is essential to comprehend the physical symptoms and implications. To reduce discomfort and avoid consequences, it is crucial to recognize it early and take proper action.

• **Emotional and Psychological Impact:** Managing a medical problem that impacts such a delicate part of the body can have significant psychological and emotional ramifications. It's possible for people with anal fistulas to feel embarrassed, frustrated, or even anxious. Increasing understanding of these elements is essential to cultivating compassion and understanding among friends, family, and the healthcare community.

• **Social Implications:** Anal fistulas have societal ramifications that go beyond the person and affect their relationships and day-to-day activities. Open communication about their situation may be difficult for patients, which might result in isolation. A thorough knowledge of anal fistulas encourages the development of a society that is more understanding and capable of offering the required support systems.

For healthcare providers, educators, and legislators, understanding anal fistulas is essential in the larger framework of public health. Resources for early identification, efficient treatment, and continuing research may be allocated by having a thorough understanding of the condition's prevalence, risk factors, and effects.

Furthermore, encouraging a better understanding of anal fistulas adds to the larger story of de-stigmatizing health-related conversations. To foster an open and encouraging healthcare environment, candid discussions about problems that may be uncomfortable or taboo are necessary.

CHAPTER 1: ANATOMY OF THE ANAL REGION

The anal area is not an exception to the rule that the anatomy of the human body is a wonder of sophisticated structures and functions like the rest of the body. To have a complete understanding of the genesis and management of anal fistulas, it is essential to have a solid understanding of the anatomy of this region. In the course of this in-depth investigation, we will dig into the general overview of the anal canal, the structures that are involved in the production of anal fistulas, and the critical significance of anal anatomy in the treatment of fistulas.

Overview of the Anal Canal

A little section of the digestive system called the anal canal joins the rectum to the exterior of the body. The anal canal, which is located between the rectum and the anus, is essential to the body's removal of waste. Its usual length is around 4 cm, and several anatomical components surround it and support its function.

The top two-thirds and the bottom one-third make up the two sections of the anal canal. While the lowest one-third is lined with stratified squamous epithelium, which resembles skin, the top two-thirds are lined with columnar epithelium, which is comparable to the rectum. The pectinate or dentate line is the name given to this transition zone.

For continence to be maintained, the muscles around the anal canal are essential. To regulate the transit of feces, two sphincters collaborate: the external anal sphincter (EAS) and the internal anal sphincter (IAS). Skeletal muscle makes up the voluntary EAS, whilst smooth muscle makes up the involuntary IAS.

Structures Involved in Anal Fistula Formation

An infection in the anal glands is usually the cause of anal fistulas. Gaining knowledge of the intricate web of glands, ducts, and tissues around the anal canal is necessary to comprehend the structures implicated in the creation of anal fistulas.

- Anal Glands: Located inside the lining of the anal canal, the anal glands are also referred to as crypts or sinuses. When it comes to lubricating the anal canal during bowel motions, these glands are essential. On the other hand, an abscess may form if an anal gland gets clogged or diseased.

- Abscess Formation: Static secretions from a clogged anal gland provide an ideal environment for bacteria to proliferate and cause an infection. An abscess, or accumulation of pus in the tissues around the anal canal, can develop from this illness.

- Tract Formation: The stored pus looks for a way out if the abscess does not drain adequately. The body naturally creates a tract, or tunnel, to link the abscess site to the skin surface close to the anus. An anal fistula is the term used to describe this tube.

Importance of Anal Anatomy in Fistula Treatment

A substantial amount of significance is placed on the complicated anatomy of the anal area when it comes to the treatment of anal fistulas. To develop beneficial treatment procedures, it is vital to recognize the role that particular structures play and the tasks that they perform. Let's take a more in-depth look at the relevant aspects:

Identification of Fistula Paths: Accurately identifying the pathways of fistulas requires an understanding of anal anatomy. To design suitable procedures, surgeons and other medical experts must comprehend the course and depth of the fistula tract.

Maintenance of Sphincter Function: When treating fistulas, maintaining sphincter function is crucial. Continence is aided by the anal sphincters, particularly the internal sphincter. By balancing the maintenance of fecal continence with efficient fistula therapy, surgical methods seek to limit harm to these sphincters.

- Stratification of Fistula Forms: There are differences in the anatomical considerations for various types of anal fistulas. The choice of treatment strategy is influenced by the classification of a fistula as intersphincteric, transsphincteric, suprasphincteric, or extrasphincteric. This in-depth knowledge makes it easier to customize therapies to the unique aspects of each situation.

- Recurrence Prevention: Recurrence of fistulas can be avoided with a thorough understanding of anal anatomy. During therapy, surgeons might address possible origins of infection, such as disease of the anal glands. Recurrence risk reduction requires anatomical identification and treatment of relevant variables.

- Patient Information and Well-Informed Choices: Patients are more empowered to take an active role in their treatment when they are informed about the anatomical features of their illness. A thorough awareness of the pertinent anatomy facilitates informed decision-making about available treatments, possible dangers, and anticipated results.

CHAPTER 2: CAUSES AND RISK FACTORS

The formation of anal fistulas is the result of a complicated interaction between several different elements, which includes widespread causes as well as particular risk factors. To have a better understanding of the genesis and probable predispositions of this ailment, patients and healthcare professionals alike need to have a solid grasp of these components. During this in-depth investigation, we will investigate the disorders that are frequently related to the creation of anal fistulas, as well as the common causes of anal fistulas, as well as the risk factors that are associated with their development.

Common Causes of Anal Fistulas

1. Anal Abscess: The development of an anal abscess is one of the main causes of anal fistulas. Pus builds up in the anal area as a result of diseased anal glands, which frequently cause abscesses. An anal fistula may develop from an abscess that is not sufficiently drained, developing into a tract or tunnel.

2. IBD (Inflammatory Bowel Disease): Disorders including Crohn's disease and ulcerative colitis, which are grouped under the term IBD, can be factors in the development of anal fistulas. Anus and rectum inflammation, in particular, raise the

risk of abscess formation and the subsequent development of a fistula in the gastrointestinal system.

3. Bacterial or viral infections in the anal area have the potential to clog the anal glands and cause an abscess to develop. Additionally linked to the development of anal fistulas are sexually transmitted illnesses like herpes or syphilis.

4. Trauma or Damage: Anal fistulas can develop as a result of trauma or injury to the anal area, which can occur from childbirth, anal surgery, or other mishaps. Anal gland damage or injury to the surrounding tissues

may set off a series of events that result in the formation of an abscess and a fistula.

5. Foreign Body Presence: When foreign bodies are present in the anal canal, it can lead to irritation, infection, and the eventual development of an abscess. Retained items or substances that don't belong in the anal tract naturally may fall under this category.

6. Diverticular disease: The lining of the digestive tract may develop tiny pouches called diverticula. Diverticula infections, especially in the rectum or anus, can cause abscesses to form and, eventually, anal fistulas too.

Risk Factors for Developing Anal Fistulas

To determine who may be more prone to anal fistulas, it is essential to comprehend the risk factors linked to this ailment. Certain risk factors can be changed, while others are innate and need to be closely managed.

- Gender: Anal fistulas are often more common in men than in women. Although the exact causes of this gender gap are unknown, variations in morphology and hormonal factors may play a role.

- Age: Although anal fistulas can develop in people of any age, young to middle-aged individuals are more likely to experience them. The occurrence of underlying illnesses, dietary habits, and lifestyle choices may all have an impact on age-related trends.

- Inflammatory Bowel Illness (IBD): Anal fistulas are considerably more common in people with inflammatory bowel disease, especially Crohn's disease. Abscesses and fistulas can occur as a result of the persistent inflammation linked to these illnesses.

- Immunosuppression: Diseases like HIV/AIDS or some drugs that weaken the immune system might make a person more vulnerable to infections. Anal abscesses might more easily grow into fistulas due to weakened immune systems.

- Diarrhea or Constipation: Prolonged intestinal problems, either with diarrhea or constipation, might aggravate the development of anal fistulas. Conditions that are favorable to the formation of an abscess might be created by straining during bowel movements or often irritating the anal canal.

- Anal Intercourse: Having anal sex without using the right lubricant or taking safety measures can cause harm to the anal area, which raises the possibility of anal fistulas. To reduce this danger, safe procedures and communication are crucial.

Conditions Associated with Anal Fistula Formation

- Crohn's Disease: There is a strong correlation between the development of an anal fistula and Crohn's disease, a chronic inflammatory disorder that can affect any region of the digestive system. Abscesses and fistulas develop as a result of the inflammation and tissue destruction that are inherent to Crohn's disease.

- The colon and rectum are the main organs affected by ulcerative colitis, another kind of inflammatory bowel disease. Anal fistulas can emerge in people with ulcerative colitis when they experience abscesses in the anal area.

- Mycobacterium tuberculosis is an infectious illness that causes TB, which can damage the anal area and lead to the formation of fistulas. This is more typical in areas where TB is endemic.

- Hidradenitis Suppurativa: This is a long-term skin disorder marked by the development of nodules and painful abscesses. These abscesses can result in the formation of anal fistulas when they happen in the perianal area.

- Diabetes: If left unchecked, diabetes can weaken the immune system and increase a person's risk of developing an abscess. People with diabetes may be more likely to develop anal fistulas, particularly if their illness is poorly treated.

- Radiation Therapy: Those who have had pelvic radiation therapy, frequently as a component of cancer treatment, may sustain tissue damage around the anus. Anal fistula formation may be facilitated by this injury.

CHAPTER 3: TYPES OF ANAL FISTULAS

The process of classifying anal fistulas is a complex one that takes into account several different aspects. These aspects include the intricacy of the fistula tract, the involvement of anatomical structures, and the possibility of recurrence. In the course of this in-depth investigation, we shall investigate the many varieties of anal fistulas, which range from straightforward to intricate variants. When it comes to developing successful treatment plans and determining the prognosis of the ailment, having a solid understanding of these categories is quite necessary.

Simple vs. Complex Fistulas

- **Simple Fistulas:**

An internal opening within the anal canal is connected to an exterior opening in the perianal skin in a straightforward and single-track tunnel that is characteristic of simple anal fistulas. This tunnel runs from the anal canal to the perianal skin. The majority of the time, these fistulas require a modest level of intricacy and may be more amenable to uncomplicated surgical techniques.

- **Complex Fistulas:**

In contrast, complex anal fistulas are characterized by the presence of several tracts, branching patterns, or higher levels of engagement with the structures that are located in the surrounding area. Both in terms of therapy and terms of the likelihood of recurrence, they frequently present a bigger challenge than other types of cancer. Complex fistulas can spread beyond the anal sphincters, which makes it more difficult to maintain continence.

Intersphincteric, Transsphincteric, Suprasphincteric, and Extrasphincteric Fistulas

The internal and external anal sphincters include intersphincteric fistulas, which are restricted inside them. The external entrance of these fistulas is typically seen in close proximity to the anal verge. The tract involved in these fistulas passes through the gap between the two sphincters. Even though these fistulas may appear less complicated, therapy must take into account their closeness to the sphincters to prevent harm to these muscles.

Transsphincteric Fistulas: These fistulas pass through the external and internal sphincters of the anus. Usually, the tract starts in the anal canal, passes through both sphincters and finishes in the perianal area. Maintaining fecal continence while managing trans-sphincteric fistulas necessitates a careful balance between curative measures and sphincter function preservation.

Suprasphincteric Fistulas: A tract that extends above the external anal sphincter is involved in these more complicated fistulas. The levator ani muscle, which is located above the sphincters, may allow this kind of fistula to flow through it. Suprasphincteric fistulas are complicated lesions that provide difficulties for both diagnosis and management.

Extrasphincteric Fistulas: Of these classifications, extrasphincteric fistulas are the most complicated. These fistulas frequently take a lengthy detour via the surrounding tissues, avoiding both the external and internal anal sphincters. Treatment may be more difficult if the tract extends into the pelvic cavity. Maintaining sphincter function is still crucial for the treatment of extra sphincteric fistulas.

Horseshoe Fistulas and Other Variations

- Horseshoe Fistulas: This particular variety is distinguished by a single external entrance surrounded by tracts that extend in both directions, creating the appearance of a horseshoe around the anus. Since these fistulas frequently spread deeper into the tissues, addressing their intricate branching pattern during surgery requires careful planning.

- High fistulas: High fistulas are defined as those that extend into the pelvic or rectal area and are typically located at a considerable distance from the anal margin. These fistulas could have a longer path through the tissues, necessitating a careful diagnosis and course of care.

- Blind-End Fistulas: These fistulas are caused by fistulas that lack an external entrance. To avoid problems, therapy for these fistulas entails locating and treating the hidden tract, which can be difficult to detect.

- Fistulas that Recur or Persist: Although not a separate kind, the persistence of fistulas following the first treatment is a crucial factor to take into account. Due to scarring from prior procedures and the requirement for meticulous planning to prevent additional recurrence, recurrent fistulas may offer difficulties.

CHAPTER 4: SYMPTOMS AND DIAGNOSIS

Anal fistulas, even though they frequently cause discomfort and cause for concern, are amenable to successful management if they are diagnosed early and accurately. First and first, to seek the right medical assistance, it is necessary to recognize the symptoms that are connected with anal fistulas. During this in-depth investigation, we will delve into the primary symptoms that are indicative of anal fistulas, emphasize the significance of early diagnosis, and talk about the diagnostic procedures that are involved, which include a physical examination, imaging techniques, and specialized tests.

Recognizing Symptoms of Anal Fistulas

Pain and Discomfort: Anal fistulas are distinguished by chronic pain and discomfort in the anal or perianal area. This discomfort can range in severity from slight soreness to severe pain, and it may worsen after bowel motions.

- Perianal Swelling: One of the most prevalent symptoms of anal fistulas is swelling around the anus. This swelling is frequently accompanied by soreness and can be seen both outwardly and internally.

- Anal fistulas usually generate a discharge that is pus-like, crimson, or purulent. The presence of discharge indicates an improper connection between the anal canal and the epidermis.

- Anal fistulas may cause inflammation and redness in the perianal region. This inflammation is typically caused by the body's reaction to the infection and can add to the overall pain felt by those with fistulas.

- Itching or discomfort around the anus can be a subsequent sign of anal fistulas. Continuous discharge and inflammation can cause skin irritation, which contributes to unpleasant symptoms.

- Fever and General Malaise: In certain situations, people with anal fistulas may develop systemic symptoms including fever and malaise. These symptoms suggest an underlying infection and may lead people to seek medical assistance.

It's crucial to keep in mind that each person may experience symptoms differently in terms of intensity and combination. While some people may only have mild discomfort, others may experience more severe symptoms. It is essential to identify these symptoms and consider how they could affect daily functioning to receive prompt medical assistance.

Importance of Early Diagnosis

- Prevention of Problems: Preventing complications from anal fistulas is mostly dependent on early detection. If left untreated, fistulas can develop into abscesses, become chronically infected, and perhaps spread to neighboring tissues. Intervention in good time can help reduce these hazards.

- Preserving Sphincter Function: When treating anal fistulas, maintaining the function of the anal sphincter is crucial. Aiming to treat the fistula while causing the least amount of harm to the sphincters, early detection enables therapies that support the maintenance of fecal continence.

- Pain and Discomfort Can Be Reduced: Anal fistulas can be treated to reduce pain and discomfort by starting therapy early on. Early in the course of the disease, focused therapies and pain management techniques are more beneficial.

- Improved Quality of Life: People with anal fistulas have a higher quality of life when they receive early diagnosis and suitable treatment. When symptoms are treated early on and problems are avoided, people can return to their regular activities without being limited by chronic pain.

Diagnostic Procedures: Physical Examination, Imaging, and Tests

Physical Examination:

The first stage in the diagnosis of anal fistulas is a complete physical assessment. To detect external openings, edema, and indications of inflammation, medical professionals including colorectal specialists may visually examine the perianal area. To examine the state of the anal canal and to assess internal openings, a digital rectal examination (DRE) may also be conducted.

Imaging Techniques:

Endoanal Ultrasound:

A useful imaging method that offers fine-grained pictures of the anal canal and its surroundings is endoanal ultrasonography. It is very helpful for determining the depth and path of the fistula tract as well as for viewing the internal fistula apertures.

Magnetic Resonance Imaging (MRI):

An additional imaging modality used to assess anal fistulas is magnetic resonance imaging (MRI). In addition to offering high-resolution pictures, it can give important details on the fistula's architecture, sphincter involvement, and any related abscesses.

Specialized Tests:

Fistulogram:

To see the path and features of the fistula, a fistulogram entails injecting a contrast dye into the fistula tract and then imaging. Making decisions and preparing treatments can be aided by this exam.

Computed Tomography (CT) Scan:

A CT scan is less frequently used to diagnose anal fistulas, although it can be performed in some circumstances to determine the level of infection and rule out consequences.

Diagnostic Tests:

Colonoscopy:

To rule out underlying diseases such as inflammatory bowel disease that may have a role in the formation of anal fistulas, a colonoscopy may be conducted. It makes it possible to examine the colon and rectum directly.

Blood Tests:

A complete blood count (CBC) and inflammatory markers are two blood tests that may be used to determine if systemic inflammation and infection are present.

Pus Culture:

It may be possible to identify the precise bacteria causing the illness by cultivating the pus from the fistula discharge. Antibiotic treatment can be guided by this information.

CHAPTER 5: UNDERSTANDING THE TREATMENT OPTIONS

A variety of surgical and medicinal procedures are used in the complex process of treating anal fistulas. The kind and intricacy of the fistula, the existence of underlying medical issues, and the specific needs of each patient all influence the treatment option. We will examine the many approaches to treating anal fistulas in this thorough analysis, including medicinal therapy, surgical procedures, and cutting-edge treatments that are still being developed in the field of colorectal medicine.

Medical Management: Antibiotics, Pain Management

1. Antibiotics:

- *Role in Infection Control:*

Antibiotics are essential for the treatment of anal fistulas, especially in cases when an infection is present. They are recommended to prevent and eliminate bacterial development in the tissues around the fistula tract.

- *Complementary to Surgical Interventions:*

Antibiotics are occasionally used in conjunction with surgical procedures. They can be given either surgically to limit recurrence or preoperatively to lessen the severity of the illness.

2. Pain Management:

- *Topical Analgesics:*

Anal fistula-related local pain and discomfort may be managed with topical analgesics, such as lidocaine ointments. These drugs work by numbing the afflicted region, which can bring relief.

- *Oral Pain Medications:*

To control pain, doctors may prescribe oral painkillers, such as nonsteroidal anti-inflammatory medicines (NSAIDs) and, in certain situations, harsher analgesics. These drugs can lessen pain and regulate inflammation.

Surgical Interventions: Fistulotomy, Fistulectomy, Seton Placement

1. Fistulotomy:

- *Procedure Overview:*

A typical surgical method for treating uncomplicated anal fistulas is a fistulotomy. The fistula tract is completely cut open by the surgeon during a fistulotomy, enabling the wound to heal internally. This method works well for simple, straight fistulas.

- *Indications and Considerations:*

Usually, fistulotomy is advised for low-profile and superficial fistulas. The distance between the fistula tract and the anal sphincters must be evaluated since injury to these muscles may affect the ability to pass stool.

2. Fistulectomy:

- *Procedure Overview:*

A fistulectomy entails the fistula tract's total removal. Fistulectomy excises the whole tract, decreasing the chance of recurrence, in contrast to fistulotomy, which opens the tract.

- *Indications and Considerations:*

Certain forms of fistulas are good candidates for fistulectomy, particularly if they are simple and clearly defined. When the preservation of the anal sphincters is the main priority, this method can be used.

3. Seton Placement:

- *Procedure Overview:*

The process of placing a seton entails passing a thin, flexible thread or tube into the fistula tract. The goal of this surgery is to keep the tract open so that it may gradually mend and drain.

- *Indications and Considerations:*

Fistulas that are difficult to treat or have a high likelihood of recurrence are frequently candidates for seton insertion. It aids in the treatment of drainage, the management of infection, and the prevention of the development of new abscesses.

4. Advanced Procedures:

- *LIFT (Ligation of Intersphincteric Fistula Tract):*

To stop the fistula's progression, a specialist technique called LIFT involves ligating the intersphincteric fistula tract. This method seeks to promote healing with the least amount of sphincter injury possible, making it appropriate for some forms of fistulas.

- Advancement Flap:

During advancement flap surgeries, the internal fistula hole is covered by adjacent tissue. This method aids in the closure of the fistula tract and healing.

Emerging Therapies: Biologics, Fibrin Sealants

1. Biologics:

- *Introduction and Mechanism:*

A class of drugs known as biologics is made from live cells. Certain biologics target particular inflammatory pathways linked to diseases such as Crohn's disease, which is frequently linked to the production of anal fistulas, in the setting of anal fistulas.

- *Indications and Considerations:*

When anal fistulas form as a result of underlying inflammatory bowel illness, such as Crohn's disease, biologics may be taken into consideration. These drugs try to lessen inflammation and regulate the immune system.

2. Fibrin Sealants:

- *Application in Fistula Treatment:*

Fibrin sealants are biological adhesives that can be used to plug fistulas' interior apertures. The goal of this method is to seal off the fistula tract to facilitate healing.

- *Indications and Considerations:*

Fibrin sealants might be used in addition to surgery, particularly when preserving continence is crucial. They may be especially helpful in cases of intricate fistulas.

Postoperative Care and Complications

1. Postoperative Care:

- *Wound Management:*

After surgery, wound care must be administered appropriately. This entails cleaning the region, taking sitz baths, and changing the dressing following the surgeon's instructions.

- *Monitoring for Infection:*

It's critical to check for infections after surgery. If an infection develops, further antibiotic medication could be advised.

2. Potential Complications:

- *Recurrence:*

Anal fistulas can reoccur, particularly if problems arise during the healing process or if the original therapy does not address underlying reasons.

- *Fecal Incontinence:*

Damage to the anal sphincters during surgery can result in fecal incontinence. Surgeons take great care to minimize this risk, but it remains a consideration, especially in complex cases.

CHAPTER 6: PREPARING FOR TREATMENT

For those who are living with this problem, the time when they are confronted with the possibility of receiving treatment for anal fistulas can be a critical occasion. It is essential to adequately prepare oneself, both emotionally and physically, to make the treatment process go more smoothly and to maximize the likelihood of successful recovery. In this all-encompassing guide, we will dig into the most important components of getting ready for treatment. We will discuss preoperative examinations, adjustments in lifestyle that can help with recovery, and the significance of becoming mentally and emotionally ready.

Preoperative Assessment

1. Consultation with Healthcare Professionals:

- Gastroenterologists and Colorectal Surgeons: Before beginning therapy, patients with anal fistulas usually have in-depth discussions with gastroenterologists and colorectal surgeons. These experts evaluate the kind and degree of the fistula, take underlying medical issues into account, and customize a treatment plan to meet the needs of the patient.

- Anesthesiologist: Should surgery be advised, the anesthesiologist will evaluate the patient's general health to choose the best anesthetic technique for the operation. This includes going over past medical records, present prescriptions, and any known allergies.

- Nursing and Support Personnel: People can better understand the treatment process, what to anticipate before and after a procedure, and how to take care of themselves while recovering by interacting with nursing and support staff.

2. Diagnostic Tests and Imaging:

- Endoanal Ultrasound and MRI: To get precise pictures of the anal canal and its surrounding tissues, diagnostic procedures like endoanal ultrasound or MRI may be performed. Surgeons can detect any problematic problems and arrange a therapeutic approach with the aid of these imaging examinations.

- Blood Tests: To evaluate the person's general health and identify any indications of infection or inflammation, routine blood tests, such as a complete blood count (CBC) and inflammatory markers, may be requested.

- Colonoscopy: If the fistula is linked to underlying illnesses such as inflammatory bowel disease, a colonoscopy, if not performed earlier, may be advised to rule them out.

3. Reviewing Treatment Options:

- Talk about Surgical Procedures: Surgeons will talk about the particular process that is advised for patients having surgical procedures, such as a fistulotomy, fistulectomy, seton placement, or other cutting-edge methods. Comprehending the selected methodology is vital for making well-informed choices.

- Examining Non-Surgical Options: When non-surgical procedures or novel therapies such as biologics are being contemplated, medical experts will furnish comprehensive details regarding these options, encompassing their possible advantages and disadvantages.

4. Clearing Doubts and Questions:

- Open Communication: People are welcome to express any worries they may have regarding the suggested course of therapy as well as to ask questions. People feel more empowered in their healthcare journey when they have open lines of contact with healthcare practitioners.

- Before undergoing any operation, patients will be asked to give informed permission, which certifies that they are aware of the possible risks, the nature of the therapy, and the anticipated results. Patients are guaranteed active participation in the decisions about their treatment through this official procedure.

Lifestyle Changes for Better Recovery

1. Nutrition and Hydration:

- A well-balanced, nutrient-dense diet is crucial for promoting the body's healing process. Adequate protein intake is especially important for tissue healing. A consultation with a nutritionist may be advantageous for tailored dietary suggestions.

- Hydration: Staying hydrated is essential for general health and can aid with recuperation. Individuals should consume adequate amounts of water and other hydrating drinks.

2. Bowel Management:

- Fiber-Rich Diet: Following anal fistula surgery, constipation might be a problem. However, a diet rich in fiber encourages regular bowel movements and helps avoid it. Whole grains, legumes, fruits, and vegetables are examples of foods high in fiber.

- Stool Softeners: To facilitate bowel movements and lessen discomfort during the postoperative phase, stool softeners or moderate laxatives may be advised. It's crucial to heed medical advice from your physician when using these drugs.

3. Physical Activity:

- Gentle Activities: Walking and moderate stretching are two examples of gentle exercises that can improve general well-being, avoid stiffness, and increase circulation. People should refrain from demanding activities that might put stress on the surgical site, nevertheless.

- Gradual Increase in Activity: Following surgery, it is usually recommended that patients increase their level of activity gradually, beginning with short walks and increasing as tolerated. This promotes the healing process and helps avoid problems.

4. Wound Care:

- Cleanliness Practices: Proper hygiene in the anal region is critical for infection prevention. After bowel motions, use gentle soap and water to clean the area and soft, non-irritating toilet paper to avoid irritation.

- Sitz Baths: Sitting in warm water can give relief while also promoting hygiene. This therapy is frequently suggested following surgery to reduce pain and promote wound healing.

Mental and Emotional Preparation

1. Understanding Emotional Impact:

- Acknowledging Feelings: Living with a medical illness and receiving treatment can elicit a variety of feelings, such as worry, fear, and frustration. Recognizing these sensations is a vital step in mental and emotional preparedness.

- Open Communication: Discussing emotional issues with healthcare practitioners, family members, or friends can give a helpful outlet. Mental health specialists may be sought for extra advice and assistance.

2. Setting Realistic Expectations:

- Treatment Outcome Expectations: While healthcare practitioners strive for the best possible outcomes, it is critical to have realistic expectations regarding the treatment process and potential problems. Discussing expected outcomes and probable issues with the healthcare team might help people psychologically prepare.

- Recovery Period: Understanding the anticipated timeline for recovery is critical for controlling expectations. Individuals should be informed that rehabilitation is a lengthy process, and healing times may differ.

3. Building a Support System:

- Family and Friends: Creating a network of family and friends may give emotional support as well as practical aid during the rehabilitation process. Communicating needs and asking for assistance when required leads to a more favorable experience.

- Support Groups: Joining a support group or interacting with others who have gone through similar treatments can bring useful insights and experiences. Online forums or local support groups organized by healthcare practitioners can be valuable tools.

4. Coping Strategies:

- Mindfulness and relaxation practices, such as deep breathing or meditation, can help you cope with stress and anxiety. These strategies can be especially useful during the preoperative phase.

- Positive Affirmations: Using positive affirmations and having an optimistic mentality will help you build resilience and cope with the obstacles of therapy.

CHAPTER 7: SURGICAL PROCEDURES IN DETAIL

Anal fistulas are often treated with surgical intervention, which is a method that is both common and successful. A number of considerations, including the kind and degree of difficulty of the fistula, the existence of underlying disorders, and the individual's overall state of health, all play a role in determining the surgical technique that should be performed. Within the scope of this in-depth investigation, we will investigate three primary surgical procedures for anal fistulas. These procedures are fistulotomy, seton placement, and advanced procedures such as LIFT (Ligation of Intersphincteric Fistula Tract), advancement flap, and the utilization of fibrin sealants.

Fistulotomy: Procedure and Recovery

Procedure:

A popular surgical method used to treat uncomplicated anal fistulas is fistulotomy. By creating an open tract, a fistulotomy aims to enable internal healing of the fistula. During the operation, an incision is made from the exterior hole in the perianal skin to the internal opening within the anal canal.

1. Preoperative Preparation:

Individuals go through a comprehensive preoperative evaluation before the treatment, which includes visits with colorectal surgeons and diagnostic examinations including MRIs and endoanal ultrasounds.

Understanding the process, its expected results and any hazards requires open communication with the medical team.

2. Anesthesia and Incision:

General anesthesia is usually used during fistulotomy procedures to guarantee the patient's comfort.

The whole fistula tract is exposed when the surgeon makes an incision from the internal to the exterior orifice.

3. Tract Exploration and Debridement:

Examining the fistula tract, the surgeon removes any debris or granulation tissue. Debridement is necessary to encourage appropriate recovery.

4. Wound Closure:

The surgeon may decide to use sutures to partially or seal the incision in some situations, or he may leave it open to heal over time.

5. Postoperative Care:

Taking good care of one's wounds during recovery entails maintaining cleanliness and refraining from activities that might put stress on the surgical site.

Pain control techniques, such as using sitz baths and prescription analgesics, can assist reduce discomfort following surgery.

6. Diet and Bowel Management:

The healing process is aided by a nutritious diet and enough water. To avoid constipation and straining during bowel movements, it's common advice to consume meals high in fiber and use stool softeners.

7. Follow-up Appointments:

To promote the best possible recovery, follow-up consultations with healthcare specialists are planned regularly to monitor the healing process and treat any issues.

Recovery:

- While recovery from a fistulotomy differs from person to person, it usually entails a gradual resumption of regular activities.

- After the operation, most people can resume mild activities quickly. Over time, they can gradually raise their physical activity levels.

- Follow-up visits enable medical professionals to monitor the healing process and handle any issues or problems that may develop.

Seton Placement: Types and Indications

Procedure:

A tiny, flexible thread or tube called a "seton" is inserted into the fistula tract during a surgical procedure called "seton implantation." The seton is meant to stay in place so that the fistula may slowly drain and mend. For difficult fistulas or those with a high risk of recurrence, seton implantation is frequently used.

1. Preoperative Assessment:

Patients have a preoperative evaluation that includes diagnostic imaging and discussions with colorectal surgeons to ascertain the kind and degree of the fistula.

2. Anesthesia and Seton Insertion:

Depending on the circumstances of each case, either local or general anesthesia is usually used for the treatment.

By inserting the seton via the fistula tract, the surgeon makes it possible for it to stay in place for a long time.

3. Types of Setons:

The purpose of a cutting seton is to gently sever the fistula tract over time. When maintaining sphincter function is important or the tract is complicated, this kind of seton is used.

Drainage Seton: To enable constant drainage of the fistula, a drainage seton is a non-cutting seton. To encourage healing and stop pus buildup in complicated fistulas, this kind of seton is frequently utilized.

4. Periodic Adjustments:

The seton may occasionally be tightened or modified to allow for a more progressive incision across the fistula tract.

5. Postoperative Care:

Following seton placement, recovery necessitates routine follow-up consultations to evaluate the healing process and monitor the seton.

Following postoperative care recommendations, maintaining good cleanliness, and managing pain are essential for a full recovery.

Indications:

Complex fistulas, those linked to illnesses like Crohn's disease, or instances with a high risk of recurrence should be treated by seton implantation.

The seton's drainage facilitates slow healing, inhibits the development of new abscesses, and aids in infection management.

Advanced Procedures: LIFT, Advancement Flap, Fibrin Sealants

1. LIFT (Ligation of Intersphincteric Fistula Tract):

Procedure:

A sophisticated surgical method called LIFT is applied to some kinds of anal fistulas, especially those that affect the intersphincteric area. To stop the fistula's progression, the intersphincteric fistula tract is ligated during the surgery.

Preoperative Assessment:

To ascertain their appropriateness for the LIFT operation, patients go through a comprehensive preoperative evaluation that includes consultations with colorectal surgeons and diagnostic imaging.

Anesthesia and Ligation:

The process is usually carried out while under general anesthesia.

The intersphincteric fistula tract is located and its continuity is broken by the surgeon by ligating it.

Advantages of LIFT:

The goal of LIFT is to lower the risk of postoperative incontinence while maintaining sphincter function.

Certain complicated fistulas that cross the intersphincteric space could benefit from this surgery.

2. Advancement Flap:

Procedure:

During advancement flap surgeries, the internal fistula hole is covered by adjacent tissue. Promoting healing and sealing the fistula tract are the objectives.

Preoperative Assessment:

The choice to perform an advancement flap operation is guided by a comprehensive preoperative examination that takes into account variables including the location and kind of fistula.

Anesthesia and Flap Advancement:

The process is usually carried out while under general anesthesia.

Using adjacent tissue, the surgeon forms a flap that is advanced to cover the fistula's internal entrance.

Advantages of Advancement Flap:

Certain fistula types are suited for advancement flap surgeries, particularly those with a well-defined internal opening.

By using local tissue, the risks associated with more involved surgical methods are mitigated.

3. Fibrin Sealants:

Procedure:

Fibrin sealants are biological adhesives that can be used to plug fistulas' interior apertures. The goal of this method is to seal off the fistula tract to facilitate healing.

Preoperative Assessment:

When preserving continence is a top concern, fibrin sealants may be used as an adjuvant to surgical operations.

Application of Fibrin Sealant:

To close up the internal fistula hole and encourage healing, the surgeon adds fibrin sealant.

Advantages of Fibrin Sealants:

Fibrin sealants have the potential to be very useful in the treatment of complicated fistulas, where the preservation of sphincter function is of utmost importance.

In addition to avoiding harm to the tissues that are nearby, the purpose of this method is to lessen the likelihood of a recurrence.

Postoperative Care and Complications

- **Postoperative Care:**

In the aftermath of surgical procedures, it is critical to provide appropriate wound care. This entails maintaining a clean environment, making use of sitz baths, and according to the advice of the surgeon about the frequency of dressing changes.

It is essential to keep an eye out for any indications of infection. If an infection develops, further antibiotic treatment can be recommended.

- **Potential Complications:**

Recurrence: Anal fistulas can occur again, particularly if the underlying reasons are not addressed by the initial therapy or if the healing process is complicated.

Fecal Incontinence: Fecal incontinence can arise from surgery-related damage to the anal sphincters. Although surgeons make great efforts to reduce this danger, it is nevertheless something to be considered, particularly in complex instances.

CHAPTER 8: POSTOPERATIVE CARE AND COMPLICATIONS

The postoperative phase is extremely important for maintaining good healing and limiting problems, even though surgery for anal fistulas is a big step towards recovery (and recovery in general). In this all-encompassing guide, we will discuss the most important parts of postoperative care, such as the management of pain and discomfort, the care of wounds and hygiene habits, and the management of any problems that may occur throughout the process of recovery.

Managing Pain and Discomfort

1. Prescribed Medications:

After anal fistula surgery, pain and suffering may vary from person to person. An essential component of postoperative treatment is pain control.

To relieve pain, take prescribed painkillers as prescribed by the doctor, such as stronger analgesics or nonsteroidal anti-inflammatory medicines (NSAIDs).

2. Topical Analgesics:

For limited comfort, topical analgesics such as lidocaine ointments could be advised. These can be used to numb the skin and reduce discomfort in the perianal region.

3. Sitz Baths:

Sitz baths, in which the patient sits in warm water, have the potential to improve general comfort and ease pain. This technique promotes relaxation and calms the operative region.

4. Positioning and Rest:

In the first few days following surgery, avoiding prolonged sitting and staying in a comfortable posture might help relieve pressure on the surgical site.

Resting enough is crucial to the healing process. People are urged to refrain from physically demanding activities and allow their bodies the time they require to heal.

Wound Care and Hygiene

1. Cleaning the Surgical Site:

Optimal healing and infection prevention depend on proper wound care. It is recommended that people wash their hands after using mild soap and water to clean the surgical site.

To reduce needless friction, pat the region dry with soft, non-irritating toilet paper.

2. Sitz Baths:

Sitz baths are a good method to stay clean in addition to relieving discomfort. To maintain the perianal region clean, people might take sitz baths many times a day, particularly after bowel movements.

3. Avoiding Harsh Products:

Hygiene items with strong scents or textures should be avoided since they might irritate the surgical site. It is best to use gentle, fragrance-free soaps when recovering after surgery.

4. Use of Cushions:

When sitting, using a cushion or inflated donut might assist relieve pressure on the surgery site. This can be especially helpful in the early stages of rehabilitation.

5. Dressing Changes:

Changes in dressings may be necessary after some surgical operations. It's essential to adhere to the healthcare provider's advice on dressing changes to keep the area clean and track the healing process.

Potential Complications and How to Address Them

Infection:

Signs of Infection:

- Elevated temperature, edema, or redness near the surgery site.

- Continuous or getting greater discomfort.

- Pus or unusual outflow.

Addressing Infection:

- Notify the healthcare professional right away if any infection-related symptoms appear.

- The infection may be controlled with the prescription of antibiotics.

Bleeding:

Signs of Bleeding:

- Much blood coming from the wound.

- Stool containing blood.

Addressing Bleeding:

- Bleeding management measures include elevating the legs and gently applying pressure to the affected region.

- It's critical to get advice from the healthcare practitioner as soon as possible.

Fistula Recurrence:

Signs of Recurrence:

- Symptoms include pain, swelling, or discharge returning.

- Visual assessment of a fistula tract that has reopened.

Addressing Recurrence:

- Quickly notify the healthcare professional of any recurrence symptoms.

- To determine the severity of the recurrence, more diagnostic testing can be carried out.

Fecal Incontinence:

Signs of Incontinence:

- Unable to regulate bowel motions.

- Stool leakage.

Addressing Incontinence:

- Speaking with the healthcare professional to identify the incontinence's cause.

- Exercises for the pelvic floor or a referral to a professional may be advised in some situations.

Delayed Healing:

Signs of Delayed Healing:

- Prolonged discomfort and pain that lasts longer than anticipated after healing.
- Insufficient or sluggish wound closure.

Addressing Delayed Healing:

- Notifying the medical professional of any enduring symptoms.
- Further evaluations, such as imaging tests, might be carried out to determine the reason for the prolonged healing process.

Allergic Reactions:

Signs of Allergic Reactions:

- Puffiness, rash, or itching at the surgery site.

- Systemic signs include lightheadedness or breathing problems.

Addressing Allergic Reactions:

- If there are indications of a serious allergic response, get medical help right away.

- Notifying the healthcare practitioner about less severe allergy reactions so that they can be appropriately managed.

CHAPTER 9: LIVING WITH ANAL FISTULA

Adapting to living with an anal fistula requires a mix of long-term planning, follow-up treatment, and coping mechanisms. People with this illness frequently discover that to achieve maximum well-being, a holistic strategy that takes into account lifestyle, mental, and physical factors is necessary. We will discuss many aspects of living with anal fistula in this extensive guide, such as coping mechanisms for the difficulties it poses, long-term health maintenance issues, and the significance of monitoring and follow-up treatment.

Coping Strategies

1. Emotional Well-being:

- Recognizing Emotions: Having an anal fistula, a chronic illness, can cause a variety of feelings, such as worry, anxiety, and irritation. To effectively cope, you must first acknowledge these feelings.

- Seeking Support: Making connections with loved ones, friends, or support groups can provide you with a listening ear and a place to talk about your experiences. Resources like local support groups and internet forums run by medical professionals can be quite helpful.

- Professional Advice: Consulting therapists or counselors who specialize in mental health issues can provide coping mechanisms and other resources to help manage the psychological effects of having an anal fistula.

2. Pain Management:

- Following Recommended Pain Management Regimens: It's important to adhere to prescribed pain management regimens to minimize suffering. Open communication regarding pain levels with medical professionals guarantees that necessary modifications may be made.

- Examining Complementary Treatments: Complementary therapies including massage, acupuncture, and relaxation methods can provide help for certain people. Although these methods cannot take the place of medical therapies, they could provide further assistance.

3. Lifestyle Adjustments:

- Dietary adjustments: Including more meals high in fiber and drinking enough water will help maintain constipation and promote bowel regularity, which can ease the healing process at the surgery site.

- Physical Activity: Regularly performing mild activities might help with digestion and enhance general well-being. But people should stay away from physically demanding activities since they might make symptoms worse.

4. Building Resilience:

Mindfulness and Stress Reduction: Engaging in mindfulness and stress-reduction practices, such as meditation or deep breathing exercises, can support resilience in the face of adversity and help control stress levels.

Positive Affirmations: Keeping an optimistic attitude and using affirmations might help you see things more positively. For general well-being, it is crucial to concentrate on areas of life that go beyond the illness.

Long-term Considerations

Disease Management:

- Underlying Disorders: It is important to continue managing the primary disease if anal fistula is linked to underlying conditions such as Crohn's disease. It is advised to have regular appointments with inflammatory bowel disease experts or gastroenterologists.

- Medication Adherence: Patients should follow their doctor's recommendations while taking prescription drugs, particularly those for treating inflammatory bowel disease or avoiding recurrence. Maintaining regular contact with medical professionals is crucial for tracking the efficacy of medications.

Continued Follow-up:

- Frequent Follow-Up: It's critical to schedule follow-up visits with colorectal surgeons or other healthcare professionals to monitor the healing process, manage any difficulties, and modify treatment plans as necessary.

- Diagnostic Tests: To evaluate the condition of the anal canal and surrounding tissues, periodic diagnostic tests, such as endoanal ultrasonography or MRI, may be advised. These examinations aid in the identification of any recurrence or newly formed fistula.

Preventive Measures:

- Lifestyle Changes: Leading a healthy lifestyle, which includes stress management, regular exercise, and a balanced diet, enhances general well-being and may help avoid issues or recurrence.

- Hygiene Measures: Maintaining consistent adherence to recommended hygiene practices, such as routine cleansing with a bar of mild soap and water, will help to ward off infections and promote recovery.

Continued Coping Strategies:

- Emotional Support: Constant emotional support is necessary while dealing with a chronic illness. Having a solid support network is still essential, whether it comes from treatment, support groups, or relationships with loved ones.

- Adaptability: A crucial component of long-term management is the ability to adjust to changes and possible obstacles. Depending on how their health changes, people may need to modify some parts of their lifestyle or treatment regimen.

Follow-up Care and Monitoring

Scheduled Appointments:

- Appointments with Colorectal Surgeons: It's critical to keep checking in with colorectal surgeons to monitor the healing process of the surgery site, discuss any issues, and modify treatment plans as necessary.

- Appointments with Gastroenterologists: People with underlying medical disorders, such as Crohn's disease, should continue to see gastroenterologists regularly. These medical professionals are qualified to evaluate how the original condition is being managed overall and how that affects the repair of anal fistulas.

Diagnostic Imaging:

- MRI or Endoanal Ultrasound: To get fine-grained pictures of the anal canal and its surrounding tissues, routine diagnostic examinations like MRI or Endoanal Ultrasound may be advised. These examinations aid in identifying any recurrence or newly formed fistula indicators.

- Colonoscopy: To keep an eye on colon health and identify any changes that can affect the management of anal fistulas, people with inflammatory bowel disease may benefit from routine colonoscopies.

Patient Education:

- Comprehending Symptoms: People are more equipped to take an active role in their treatment when they receive continuing education regarding the signs and symptoms of anal fistulas, potential consequences, and the significance of early management.

- Communication with Healthcare Providers: Keeping lines of communication open and continuous with healthcare providers guarantees that new symptoms or concerns are swiftly handled. Proactively managing diseases is aided by this strategy.

Quality of Life Assessment:

- Physical and Emotional Well-Being: It is critical to evaluate and treat the effects of anal fistula on both physical and emotional well-being. During follow-up visits, healthcare practitioners may ask about areas of quality of life to customize interventions.

CHAPTER 10: PREVENTION AND LIFESTYLE CHANGES

Both the adoption of a healthy lifestyle and the prevention of the recurrence of anal fistulas are essential components of long-term care. Individuals can improve their general well-being and lower the risk of difficulties by following advice about their nutrition and lifestyle, as well as by making frequent checkups a priority. In this all-encompassing guide, we will discuss the most important methods for preventing recurrences, as well as suggestions about nutrition and lifestyle, and the need of maintaining frequent checkups for the management of anal fistula.

Preventing Recurrence

1. Addressing Underlying Conditions:

- Identification and Treatment: The best way to stop the recurrence of anal fistulas in patients with underlying illnesses like Crohn's disease is to manage the main disease well. Maintaining and improving the treatment plan for underlying diseases can be made easier with routine consultations with gastroenterologists.

- Medication Adherence: It's critical to take prescription drugs as directed, particularly those that address underlying inflammatory problems. Maintaining regular contact with medical professionals guarantees the efficacy of prescription drugs and permits necessary modifications.

2. Hygiene Practices:

- Frequent Cleaning: To minimize the risk of problems and avoid infections, it is important to maintain appropriate hygiene habits in the anal area. The perianal area may be kept clean by routinely washing it with mild soap and water, especially after bowel movements.

- Sitz Baths: It might be helpful to include sitz baths in your regimen. In addition to offering relaxation, this method improves hygiene and could help stave off illnesses.

3. Dietary Modifications:

- High-Fiber Diet: Consuming a high-fiber diet encourages regular bowel movements and helps ward off constipation. Fruits, vegetables, whole grains, and legumes are good sources of fiber. Consuming enough fiber lessens the pressure on the anal area when passing stool.

- Hydration: Maintaining adequate hydration is important for general health and can help to make stools softer and make bowel motions easier. It is advised that people continue to consume enough water and other hydrating liquids.

Dietary and Lifestyle Recommendations

1. Avoiding Trigger Foods:

- Finding Triggers: People may notice that eating particular foods makes their symptoms worse. Caffeine, spicy meals, and high dairy intake are common causes. Preventing and recognizing these triggers can help control symptoms.

- Food Diary: Keeping a food diary can assist people in seeing patterns and making educated nutritional decisions by tracking eating habits and symptoms. Having this knowledge handy while speaking with medical professionals might be beneficial.

2. Regular Exercise:

- Encouraging Bowel Regularity: Exercise regularly can help maintain regular bowel movements and improve general health. Taking part in exercises like yoga, swimming, or walking promotes intestinal health.

- Avoiding Strenuous Activities: Although exercise has many advantages, people should refrain from engaging in activities that might put stress on the surgical site. Exercise regimens that are gradual and moderate are usually advised, with modifications made depending on each person's recovery and health situation.

3. Weight Management:

- Keeping a Healthy Weight: Obesity can aggravate and precipitate several medical issues, including those that impact the anal area. A balanced diet and consistent exercise help maintain a healthy weight, which benefits general health.

- Consulting with Nutritionists: When it comes to managing weight, seeking the advice of nutritionists or dietitians can yield tailored recommendations about food selections and lifestyle adjustments.

4. Stress Management:

- Techniques for Mindfulness and Relaxation: Long-term stress can affect intestinal health. Stress levels may be managed by using mindfulness and relaxation practices like yoga, deep breathing exercises, and meditation.

- Realistic Goal-Setting: Reducing stress can be achieved by controlling expectations and establishing realistic goals. People are encouraged to discuss their worries and difficulties in an open manner with healthcare professionals.

Importance of Regular Check-ups

1. Scheduled Follow-up Appointments:

- Appointments with Colorectal Surgeons: It is important to schedule routine follow-up visits with colorectal surgeons to monitor the healing process, evaluate general health, and address any issues. Treatment regimens might be modified throughout these sessions following each patient's needs.

- Gastroenterologist Appointments: Appointments with gastroenterologists are essential for those with underlying diseases such as Crohn's disease. These medical professionals keep an eye on the primary disease's treatment and how it can affect the healing of anal fistulas.

2. Diagnostic Tests:

- Endoanal Ultrasonography or MRI: To get precise pictures of the anal canal and its surrounding tissues, routine diagnostic procedures like endoanal ultrasound or MRI may be advised. These examinations aid in the identification of any recurrence or newly formed fistula.

- Colonoscopy: To evaluate the condition of the colon and identify any changes that may affect the management of anal fistulas, people with inflammatory bowel disease may have frequent colonoscopies.

3. Quality of Life Assessment:

- Physical and Emotional Well-Being: Medical professionals may ask about a patient's quality of life at follow-up visits, taking into account both their physical and emotional health. This evaluation aids in modifying treatments to target certain issues affecting general health.

- Open Communication: Patients and their healthcare professionals can have open communication during routine examinations. This kind of cooperation encourages proactive preventative care and continuous management.

4. Education and Empowerment:

- Comprehending Symptoms: People are more equipped to take an active role in their treatment when they receive continuing education regarding the signs and symptoms of anal fistulas, potential consequences, and the significance of early management.

- Talking About Lifestyle Changes: Medical professionals may provide advice on leading a healthy lifestyle and making wise decisions. Personalized advice may be given by talking about stress management, exercise regimens, and food habits.

CONCLUSION

Treatment for anal fistulas entails a multifaceted approach that includes education, preventative care, and continuous dedication. This guide has covered all of the complex aspects of anal fistulas, including their etiology, anatomy, and potential forms and treatments. It's critical to highlight important lessons learned and stress the need for a comprehensive strategy for living with anal fistula as we draw to a close to this research.

Holistic Understanding: The path starts with a comprehensive comprehension of anal fistulas, acknowledging them as complicated disorders requiring both specialized medical knowledge and personal involvement. People who are aware of the complexities of anatomy, causes, and kinds can take an active role in choosing their course of therapy and have educated conversations with their medical professionals.

Treatment Options: Patients can get a range of treatments, from sophisticated procedures and seton installation to surgical interventions including fistulotomy and antibiotic therapy. New treatments such as fibrin sealants and biologics highlight how the healthcare environment is changing. An in-depth analysis of surgical techniques, wound management, and probable complications provides insightful information on the complex healing process.

Getting Ready for Treatment: Getting ready for treatment includes not just a preoperative evaluation but also thinking about lifestyle modifications and mental health. Individuals can effectively traverse the preparatory period by focusing on physical preparedness, adaptability, and emotional resilience through collaborative partnerships with healthcare practitioners.

Surgical Operations in Detail: The wide range of methods that are accessible is highlighted by the thorough examination of surgical procedures, which include fistulotomy, seton implantation, and sophisticated treatments like LIFT, advancement flap, and fibrin sealants.

Every surgery has particular advantages, disadvantages, and possible issues that call for a customized approach to care.

Complications and Postoperative Care: The treatment of pain, wound care, and careful observation of any complications are the main focus of postoperative care, which is an important stage in the process. A complete recovery depends on identifying and treating problems including infection, bleeding, recurrence, fecal incontinence, and delayed healing.

Living with an Anal Fistula: Coping mechanisms, long-term considerations, and the significance of follow-up treatment are all part of living with an anal fistula, which goes beyond medical procedures. A comprehensive strategy for living well with this illness includes continuing therapy, quality of life evaluation, and techniques for controlling emotions.

Prevention and Lifestyle Modifications: Treating underlying issues, upholding hygienic standards, implementing dietary adjustments, and implementing lifestyle changes are all part of preventing recurrence. Ongoing preventative efforts are based on regular check-ups, diagnostic testing, and open contact with healthcare practitioners.

A Wholesome Strategy for Long-Term Health:

In summary, managing anal fistulas calls for an all-encompassing strategy that combines medical expertise, preventative care, and personal dedication. People are urged to actively interact with their healthcare professionals, accept lifestyle alterations, and prioritize their physical and mental well-being as they navigate the difficulties of treatment, recovery, and continuing maintenance.

Through the development of a cooperative relationship between patients and healthcare professionals, we open the door to a better-educated and empowered method of managing anal fistulas. The path ahead is marked by new treatments, changing viewpoints, and a dedication to improving the lives of those with anal fistulas. The road ahead in the quest for resilience, knowledge, and well-being is one of comprehension, adjustment, and ongoing assistance.